Dr. Joel's Be Super Fit with 23Ingredients

Eat And Repeat, Twice Daily, For Health, Wealth and Happiness

Life is Like A Marathon, Train For It!

Protect Your Body Against Five Deadly Diseases

Turn On Your Longevity Genes

Self-Care Is Health Care from the Inside Out

A WHOLE BODY HEALTH SERIES

DR. JOEL "RAUCH" RAUCHWERGER M.D.

and ALEXIA PARKS

PUBLISHED BY ALEXIA PARKS 10TRAITS LEADERSHIP INSTITUTE

BOULDER, COLORADO - 10TRAITS.org

23INGREDIENTS Menu Planner and **Dr. Joel's Be Super Fit** are part of 10TRAITS.org - Whole Body Health Series with Dr. Joel "Rauch" Rauchwerger M.D. and Alexia Parks

Website: https://10TRAITS.org

1. Feeding Your Miracle Brain (DVD)
2. Unlocking the Secrets of Longevity (DVD)
3. Easy Weight Loss (DVD)
4. The New Nutrition (DVD)
5. Super HIGH Energy (DVD)
6. Tuning Up Your Digestive System (DVD)
7. How to Buy and Use Supplements (DVD)
8. Dr. Rauch's "Super" Foods (DVD)
9. A GOOD Night's Sleep (DVD)
10. Nutrition for Seniors (DVD)

Dr. Joel's BE SUPER FIT Program

Published by **Alexia Parks 10TRAITS Leadership Institute** 2019 formerly The Education Exchange (SAN #253-0872) 303-443-3697 WEB: **10TRAITS.org** Boulder, CO 80302 | alexiaparks@gmail.com

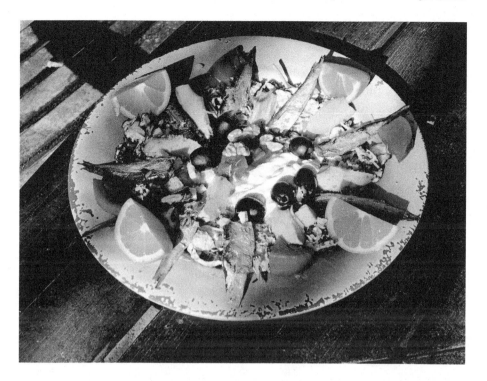

FINE DINING ON $5-A-DAY

23Ingredients to eat and repeat, twice daily, for Life, Health and Happiness.

<u>DRLONGEVITY.ORG</u>: A HEALTHY LIFESTYLE AND LONGEVITY MEAL PLANNER

Mother Nature gave us so many wonderful ingredients to enjoy, why limit yourself to just 23? Here's why: When you eat and repeat this same meal twice a day, it will both simplify your life and save you money, while lifting you to a higher level of health.

FINE DINING on $5-A-Day offers a shopping list of 23 ingredients that combine to create a 5-Star dining experience. First, it looks like a meal you might be served at the best restaurant in town.

Second, it's low cost, with off-the-shelf produce and local products that give a boost to the local economy.

Third, every bite is delicious. It offers a burst of pleasure that turns your dining experience into pure joy. I'm saying this from personal experience. As a person who has spent a lifetime dining out 80% of the time, I've now switched to dining at home, enjoying the same meal twice a day for the last 50-days.

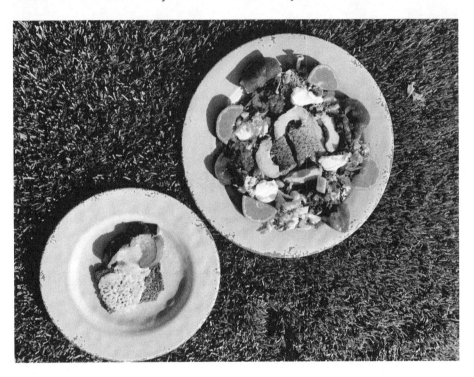

Over the years, our kitchen as been the test kitchen for Dr Joel. The FINE DINING ON $5 DAY - 23INGREDIENTS meal plan has been refined over 50-years by Dr Joel. At age 76, he hasn't been sick in 50-years, not even a common cold.Finally, after 50 years of experimentation, he has finally come up with a recipe that I love and enjoy every day, twice daily.

For me, these 23 ingredients have become **The GOLD Standard** for a good meal.

It is the meal that I compare with all other meals when dining out, and while some of these may come close for one-time pleasure, none match the power of this twice daily meal to:

1. **Help your body do "home repair" daily that includes recycling unwanted debris.**
2. **Turn on the known longevity genes. This is good!**
3. **Protect your body against five deadly diseases: high blood pressure, heart disease, diabetes, dementia and colorectal cancer.**

The food choices that make up 23Ingredients include 75% soft and hard fiber, 10% good fat and 15% protein. It's a universal, scalable meal plan.

23Ingredients single recipe shows you how to create a simple, repeatable, 5-STAR meal, served twice a day, that includes all the essential ingredients that you need to fuel a high energy lifestyle for optimum health and longevity, at the lowest possible cost using locally available foods.

It features a simple, elegant meal that your whole body will love. A twice daily meal that offers fine dining a day for two, your microbiome and you, for only pennies a day!

GETTING TO KNOW YOUR BODY:

The human body is like a car. It is constructed in a certain way so that when you turn the key on, the engine starts. A car is built on an assembly line and every thing is the same. Every part goes in the same place and has a purpose, a function.

The human body is the same. This basic recipe includes 23 ingredients - essential for whole body health - that serve as a reminder to us that LIFE thrives on consistency. The human body thrives on doing things the same way every day, regardless of circumstances.

When we try to change the Rules of Life, and introduce unexpected variables, it is like throwing sand in the gas tank, or sugar. Pay attention. Stay mindful. Use this smart little book to help you create a set of habits and stick with them to get the result you are seeking: happiness, health and longevity fueled by super high energy.

THE BOTTOM LINE:

Streamline your life. Your body thrives on consistency. Keep your food choices consistent. Keep the time of day you eat, consistent.

PRACTICE INTERMITTENT FASTING

Chose two times a day, within an 8 hour period for your two meals. Let your body fast - without food - for 12-16 hours a day.

- Eat two (2) meals a day within 8-hours. Let your body REST without food for 12-16 hours
- A resting body will automatically clean house. It will recycle & release any harmful debris daily.

FINE DINING FOR TWO: YOUR MICROBIOME AND YOU.

YOUR Body is mostly made up of protein: Your bones are 95% protein, your muscles, tendons and ligaments are protein, your sex and stress hormones require high quality protein, so do healthy hair and nails.

Your GUT is a muscle. Hard vegetables like celery, broccoli, and cauliflower act like a broom to sweep out your gut and also provide it with the daily exercise it needs for toning.

By contrast, **YOUR Microbiome** - a recently discovered 3-pound organ in your colon - loves soft fruits and vegetables. The favorite food of the 40 trillion bacteria that comprise the Microbiome is soft fruits and vegetables. When you feed them the food they love they reward you by producing 90% of the *feel good* seratonin in your body. When you feed it the soft fruits and vegetables it loves, it will also produce butyric acid.

YOUR Brain and Heart will thank your happy Microbiome for providing them with butyric acid. They both run 25% better on butyric acid.

GOOD FATS like butter, sour cream, high fat yogurt, high fat cheese, high fat cream cheese, olive oil, canola oil, avocados, coconut oil are the preferred fuel of the body. The body can burn carbohydrates and fat. Choose good fats and reap the benefits, for life.

REMEMBER to keep the skin on all fruits and vegetables. That's where the fiber is. German dark rye bread is 7% fiber. Enjoy a 2x3-inch slice.

OPTIONAL FIBER for easy weight loss: You can also buy and include 1-Tablespoon per meal of both oat BRAN (soluble fiber) and **wheat** BRAN (insoluble fiber). It is the *cap* of the grain, not the grain. This low cost addition at each meal can be used to keep you *regular* and also give you a feeling of satiety or fullness.

The food choices that make up 23INGREDIENTS include 70% soft and hard fiber, 15% good fat and 15% protein.

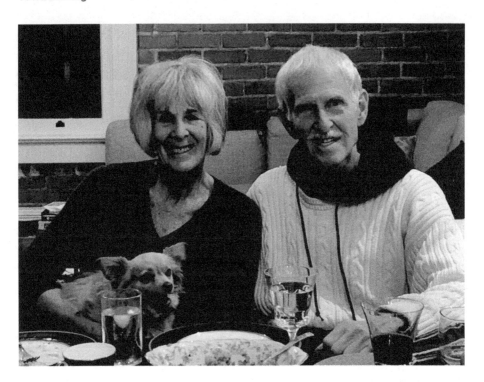

The 23Ingredients Shopping List and Menu Planner by Dr Joel and Alexia Parks (pictured above) includes:

- Ingredients for Fine Dining on $5 Day. - A meal that feeds two, your microbiome and you!

- A Weekly Shopping List based on Mother Nature. This list has been refined over 50-years by Dr Joel. At age 76, he hasn't been sick in 50-years, not even a common cold.

WHO WE ARE

Meet Dr Joel Rauch (Rauchwerger M.D.) also known as Dr Longevity and Alexia Parks - Dr Joel is a medical doctor, and an expert in whole body health and nutrition. Dr Rauch worked with well-known cardiologist and heart surgeon **Dr. Michael DeBakey** and was on the faculty at the **Baylor College of Medicine**, Houston, TX. He was also part of the team of medical doctors who worked on the case of the "**Baby in the Bubble.**" What makes Dr. Rauch unique in the field of whole body health is his vast knowledge of science, medicine, brain function, nutrition, biochemistry and psychology, as well as the fundamentals of basic, good digestion, the **micro biome**, a ketogenic lifestyle, human psychology, stress management and biofeedback. **Dr Joel has had a life long interest in how to strengthen the Immune System to prevent, reduce, or reverse most disease.**

Alexia Parks, Co-Author of 23Ingredients

Called "**One of 50 Who Matter Most on the NET**" by *Newsweek* magazine for her launch of one of the first electronic democracy websites on the Internet (1995), **Alexia Parks** is the Inventor of the Gender Equality Tool™ and a United Nations Mentor. As a UN Mentor, **Alexia Parks mentored the young leader who became the #1 Award Winner** at the Goldman Sachs/Fortune Most Powerful Woman Summit in 2014. Alexia Parks, Co-Founder of the Alexia Parks 10TRAITS Institute, based in Boulder, CO, is also the inventor of **10TRAITS™ 1-Minute Conflict Resolution Tool** and the author of 14 books. A science-writer, she formerly wrote for the national desk of *The Washington Post*. Wikipedia

WEB: DrLongevity.org | Subscribe on YouTube.com | alexiaandjoel longevity

YOUR WEEKLY SHOPPING LIST

Your GOAL is 2 MEALS a Day within 8-hours. This Gives You ALL the Health Benefits of Intermittent Fasting. Example: Lunch at 12-Noon; Dinner at 7pm

USE ALL 23 Ingredients In Each MEAL
Chose local, equivalent, fruits and vegetables

Category	CHOP, Prep and Design Ideas for Each ITEM. The Cost: **$5-A-Day** for BOTH Lunch AND Dinner	Quantity	Ingredients
GREENS Vegetable	RAW Spinach and Kale. Sliced Avocado, Onion, Garlic, Celery, Cabbage, Ginger, Dark RED Bell Pepper, Yam (Sweet Potato), Salsa	1-2 Cups Chopped Greens	9
Optional	Olives, Tomatoes, Brussel Sprouts, Mushrooms, Broccoli, Cauliflower, Bok Choy or other favorites.		4
Optional: Soluble and Insoluble Fiber Options	**1-Tablespoon** EACH for Easy Weight Loss. OAT Bran - **Soluble** fiber. This is the *cap* of the oat. 1-tablespoon of oat bran swells to 10 times its size in your GUT to give you a feeling of fullness. Wheat BRAN - **Insoluble** fiber. This is the *cap* of the wheat. It acts as a *broom* to sweep out the GUT.		2
FRUIT	Chop or Slice: Apple, Banana, Orange + Raisins	Decorate with Colorful Fruits	4
Optional	Grapefruit, Mango, Persimmon and other fiber-rich fruit.		
GOOD FAT	**OMEGA 3 (DHA & EPA) 1-TBSP Daily + High FAT:** Sour Cream, Yogurt, Butter, Nut Butter, + ONE Cheese: Brie, Havarti, Gouda, or Edam, + Olive Oil		6
Optional	Avocado, Salad Dressing made with Olive Oil and spices + Coconut Oil, 4-8 Walnuts, Chocolate Chips		4

YAM (SWEET Potato)	BUY **5-7** for the week and bake yam (sweet potatoes) at 350-degrees for 2-Hours. Then place the baked potatoes in the refrigerator. When ready to eat, take 1-2 slices, melt butter and cheese and enjoy twice daily.	1/4 - 1/2
PROTEIN	**Choose ONE Protein Per Meal: 2-EGGS, or fish** such as 1/2 of a TIN of Sardines (rated 100% protein). Other protein options include: Fish, Beef, Fish, Chicken, or other animal protein.	Chose one protein, 2 times a day
Did You Know?	Beef broth only has 8 amino acids. The protein chosen by Dr. Joel - and listed above - has all 20-amino acids.	
	Remember: You are eating for two (2): your microbiome and you. Animal PROTEIN feeds YOU. Soluble and Insoluble FIBER feeds your microbiome. **Protein from an animal** is needed for your bones, muscles, tendons, ligaments, and all of your body chemistry including your sex and stress hormones. Your microbiome is a 3-pound organ located in your GUT. It is comprised of 50-Trillion bacteria. It is one of the most complex eco-systems in the world. It reflects 1-to1 what you EAT. It produces 90% of the feel good seratonin; and butyric acid that makes your brain and heart work 25% better. Your microbiome also coats the lining of your colon to protect against colorectal cancer.	
Did You Know?	95% of your bones are made of protein. 5% is calcium.	
Remember **Your** VITAMINS	The word **Vitamin** means VITAL for LIFE. Daily vitamins should include: B, C, D-3, E, and F (Omega 3). Add calcium citrate (1G) daily, and B-12 sublingual weekly. + 1 TBSP Nutritional Yeast Flakes dissolved in 2TBSP water, daily for low cost Vitamin B.	5+

ABOUT THE AUTHORS

Dr. Joel Rauch (Rauchwerger M.D.) is a medical doctor and an expert in whole body health and nutrition. In 1973 Dr. Rauchwerger worked in the department of a well-known cardiologist and heart surgeon Dr. Michael DeBakey, and was on the faculty at the Baylor College of Medicine, Division of Experimental Biology in the Department of Surgery, Houston, Texas.

He was also part of the team of medical doctors who worked on the case of the **"Baby in the Bubble"**, the baby born without an Immune System. This event was turned into a move: *The Baby in the Bubble*, starring John Travolta.

What makes Dr. Joel unique in the field of whole-body health, is his vast knowledge of science, medicine, brain function, nutrition, biochemistry and physiology, as well as the fundamentals of basic, good digestion, human psychology, stress management and biofeedback. Because of this, he has had a life long interest in how to strengthen the Immune System to prevent, reduce or reverse most disease.

Known as Dr. Longevity, Dr. Joel is the star of a 10-DVD series on Whole Body Health, produced by Alexia Parks 10TRAITS Leadership Institute (formerly The Education Exchange). His works are available online at the DrLongevity.org bookstore. Topics range from Feeding Your Miracle Brain, and Tuning Up Your Digestive System, to How to Get a GREAT Night's Sleep, to Nutrition for Seniors.

Alexia Parks is an inspirational speaker, and the author of 14 books, including 10TRAITS Leaders of Power and Courage, 23Ingredients, Fine Dining on $5-A-Day, and *Parkinomics*, a business and motivational bestseller on amazon.com. Alexia Parks is also Founder and CEO of 10TRAITS.com and 10TRAITS Leadership Institute, a non-profit.

CONTENTS

INTRODUCTION

FOUR MAJOR THEMES RUN THROUGHOUT THIS BOOK

They include:

#1 Boost Your Immune System. The most powerful SUPER FIT mechanism is the one that Mother Nature gave us which operates around the clock. It is our precious Immune System.

#2 Reduce Stress. Stress, in all its forms and varieties, is the biggest threat to your Immune System. These include the stress of everyday life, emotional stress, and stress from environmental toxins. Even good stress has an impact.

#3 Reduce Free Radicals. Daily life itself generates free radicals. When we experience stress, from any source, this generates massive amounts of free radicals inside your body, "running loose in a china shop." In excess they can cause rapid aging. Indiscriminate, free radicals damage everything they hit, including your DNA. Damaged DNA can mutate into a cancer cell.

This book will help you learn how to use: food, spices, supplements and even visualization to help "mop-up" free radicals.

#4 Use These Techniques to Stay SUPER FIT and to prevent, reduce or reverse most diseases.

THE STORY OF FIBER

How many people remember the TV talk show host Johnny Carson? He had a guest on his program many years ago, a psychiatrist named Dr. David Rubin. Dr. Rubin had written the first popular book on sex titled *"All you Need to Know about Sex but Were Afraid to Ask."* It became a *New York Times* bestseller. It was the first to discuss sex in public before a mass television audience.

After his appearance on the Johnny Carson show, Dr. David Rubin disappeared for many years. And then, all of a sudden, he came out with a second book. The book was on fiber in the diet. So everyone wondered why is a psychiatrist who wrote a popular book on sex, writing a book on *fiber* in the diet? A book on sex? Yes. But a book on fiber? It doesn't make sense.

Well, it seems that his own Dad, age 52, had cancer of the colon. And Dr. Rubin wanted to help his Dad. So he went to the medical literature and, sure enough, the answer was right there in the medical literature, overlooked and collecting dust.

The medical article was authored by one of the most famous doctors of all time: Sir Dennis Burkitt. Who was Dr. Dennis Burkitt? Well, he was so famous that they named a lymphatic cancer after him, cancer of the lymph nodes: Burkitt's lymphoma. This, plus his other contributions, earned him a Knighthood from the British Queen.

Here is Burkitt's story. In his retirement he was traipsing through East Africa, and made a seminal observation in Kenya. What he noticed was, that because of old colonial system of government set up by the British, modern day Kenya has two groups of people: the indigenous Kenyans and descendants of the colonials.

Dr. Burkitt's amazing discovery was that the rate of colon cancer in the two populations was like night and day: black and white.

It was completely different. In the descendants of the British Colonials, the incidence of colon cancer was sky high. In the native Kenyans, it was almost zero.

Dr. Burkitt figured out that the difference was based on what they ate, or didn't eat. It was nutritional. It was because the British population, by force of culture, would eat a lot of refined, baked goods, such as tea and crumpets. By contrast, the indigenous population had huge amounts of fiber in their diet, from corn, and from many different types of vegetables, including fibrous potatoes and yams with their skin intact.

Dr. Burkitt wrote-up his results. These results were published in the medical journals; however, no one really saw them, or did anything about them, until Dr. David Rubin saw them. And Dr. Rubin, of course, wanted to help his Dad. At the time there was only one medical remedy for colon cancer: surgical removal of the colon.

However, Dr. Rubin was so impressed by what he learned through Dr. Burkitt, that he wrote a book entitled: The Save Your Life Diet.

The focus of the book was on the use of **wheat bran**, as fiber in the diet. Wheat bran is not a food, it has no calories. It is simply the outer shell of the wheat and costs less than 50-cents for a month's supply. At 1-tablespoon-a-day, that's only pennies a day. Its daily use could reduce the incidence of colon cancer. Share this with your family!

What's the connection between wheat bran and colon cancer? The short version is this: we all have approximately two pounds of bacteria living in our lower GI system, our colon. Any excess bile from the liver, which is not needed to break down or emulsify fats, makes its way to the colon on a daily basis. There, it is acted upon by those two pounds of bacteria. The bacteria will quickly turn the excess bile into a cancer producing compound called 3-Methylcholanthrene (**3MC**).

Three-Methylcholanthrene is used in medical laboratories, on a daily basis, to produce cancers in mice so they can do research on cancer in a laboratory setting.

This daily production of **3MC**, however, occurs in all people, every day, as a normal, daily, bacterial byproduct of bile in the colon.

So, the basic logic here is to eliminate the cancer producing **3MC** from the colon each day, using 1 tablespoon of wheat bran. This supports Mother Nature's need for regularity. Wheat bran supports a daily bowel movement and clears the colon of cancer producing 3MC each day.

Here is what it does inside your body. The wheat bran is insoluble, which is good. This means that it does not dissolve in water. It acts like a scouring brush to clean the mucosa, which is the lining of the colon and keep it free of 3MC.

Colon Cancer Prevention Goal: If a person takes 1 tablespoon of wheat bran per day (at a cost of around 48 cents per month) to be regular and constantly flush out the toxic cancer-producing compound **3MC** from the colon.

It's that simple! The daily addition of wheat bran to your diet does just that.

THE TYPE "C" PERSONALITY

In the 1950's two California cardiologists, Dr. Friedman and Dr. Rosenman, made a great discovery. They were the first to really show how the mind is connected to the body. They noticed that in hard-driving people, especially men who never relaxed, their incidence of heart attacks was sky high, much higher than the general population. So they coined the term "the **TYPE A** Personality", showing that on-going mental stress is reflected in the body by disease. In this case, heart attacks.

They called the relaxed person "the **TYPE B** Personality".

The mechanism would be that this hard-driving individual, with an executive type personality that never relaxes, is constantly evoking the **"stress hormone"**. Adrenalin comes from the inside of the adrenal gland. Because all hormones in the body have target tissues, **the target of adrenalin is the heart!**

In the **Type A** person, the heart is under constant attack from this **SHORT-TERM** stress. The adrenalin response is also known as the body's *flight or fight* response. This puts pressure on the heart and the entire cardio-vascular system. The blood rushes into the arms and legs for rapid response and the digestive system is shut down.

More recent medical information has discovered another stress hormone outside of the adrenal gland. This hormone is called **Cortisone**. The target tissues of cortisone is not the heart, it is the body's **IMMUNE DEFENSE SYSTEM**.

Cortisone is evoked in **long term,** chronic stress, might be referred to as the *Type C Personality - cancer personality*. So, the cortisone hormone is evoked in the **Type C** cancer personality, the long-suffering personality.

Let's quickly summarize here:

- Our stress glands are called the adrenal glands. They have TWO separate parts: an inside, and an outside.

- They produce two separate stress hormones. The hormone released from the inside of the adrenal gland causes the **short-term stress response**.

- In the **TYPE A** personality, the target tissue of the adrenalin is the heart and the cardiovascular system.

- The other hormone, **cortisone**, is evoked whenever there is long-term stress. Here, cortisone is released from the outside of the adrenal gland, called the cortex.

The psychological profile shows that the Type A personality evokes the short-term adrenaline fight or flight response. By contrast, the **TYPE C** personality, the long-suffering, chronically stressed person, will evoke the body's cortisone response. The target tissue of the hormone cortisone is the **Immune System**. [for this reason, <u>it is critical that those with a Type C personality, change their lifestyle to ensure that stress is minimized, *continuously*</u>]. As you **reduce stress** in your life, you **boost** your **Immune System**.

Simply put, the new information is that **a strong immune system is your best defense against cancer**. In all medical textbooks, the Immune System is actually referred to as the "Immune Surveillance System Against Cancer".

So it doesn't matter how the cancer arises, or is caused. A strong Immune System will check and kill cancer in the body through its thymus derived Killer T-Cells. And, medically, that's actually their name; KILLER T-Cells.

So once the cortisone hormone starts to target or compromise your body's Immune Defense System, and specifically your KILLER T-Cells, then cancers of many types will go unchecked in the body.

As a final note, the Type A personality affects more men than women because of their hard-wiring; whereas the Type C affects more women. Usually, men let out their feelings explosively, and this short-term stress hits their cardiovascular system. Women (and men) who hold in their emotions, chronically, could be said to have the Type C personality.

TUNING UP YOUR DIGESTIVE SYSTEM

As we get older, we start to get a little wrinkled. The same way that we dry out on the outside, "we dry out on the inside". For example, I don't have the same digestive juices I had when I was captain of the tennis team back in my high school days.

The good news is that we can actually put back what we have lost! This is an easy way to do it....

We have three food groups: protein, fat and carbohydrates. Similarly, we have three digestive organs that correspond to these three food groups. It's a division of labor. The **stomach** digests **protein** with hydrochloric acid. The **liver** digests fats using green bile and the **pancreas** digests **carbohydrates** with pancreatic enzymes.

As we get older, all of these digestive juices are reduced. I remember growing up at a time when the family medicine cabinet was filled with digestive aids such as Tums, Rolaids, Pepto Bismol and Alka Seltzer, and these were the non-prescription ones! Today, pharmacies and grocery stores are filled with these same digestive aids and many more.

What a lot of people don't realize is they can actually buy digestive enzymes in a non-prescription form, they are safe to use.

The digestive enzyme for the stomach is **hydrochloric acid**. In a health food store, it might be labeled [Betaine] **Hydrochloric Acid (HCL)**. For the liver, you can buy OX bile to help out with liver digestion. And for carbohydrates, you can buy pancreatic enzymes. You can buy them separately or combines, all in one.

Years ago, I wrote a little pamphlet titled: ***The Acid Test***. At the age of 60, we have already lost 60% of our digestive juices. Here's the catch: if I have acid indigestion, I don't know whether it's because I have too much stomach acid or <u>too little, because the symptoms are approximately the same</u>.

Most people, who have indigestion, especially if they are seniors, will take an antacid, such as Tums, Rolaids or Alka Seltzer.... but that's <u>the last thing</u> they should take. They should avoid depleting the precious little hydrochloric acid **HCL** in their stomach. They need strong, undiluted **HCL** to digest protein.

Strong stomach acid is needed to fully digest the protein in each meal. Undigested protein that passes out of your stomach and into your lower digestive tract is treated like a "foreign protein" by your body. Allergies can be created by foreign protein that the body does not recognize and attacks.

A word about indigestion. In microbiology, Salmonella and Shigella are two of the biggest bacterial infections that affect the body. They are often ingested as a result of eating food from a buffet that has not been properly prepared, or has not been kept hot or cold enough. One or both can cause a stomach ache, or abdominal pain. However, if you have a sufficient amount of undiluted hydrochloric acid in your stomach, it will automatically kill those bacteria as they pass through it.

Here's something else that's valuable to know. If you drink a lot of liquid with your meal — such as coffee, tea, soda, water, soup or beer — these liquids will dilute your precious hydrochloric acid. If you drink AND eat too much at any one meal, the diluted hydrochloric acid from an overly filled stomach may back up into your esophagus. That "burning sensation" that you feel is called acid reflux. Usually, it's not from having too MUCH acid but, instead, **from having too little acid**. To avoid this, **<u>drink liquids 30 minutes before or after a meal</u>**. A small amount of wine - a half a glass - with a meal is fine. It will help stimulate the flow of digestive juices.

DR JOEL'S 10 STEP BE SUPER FIT FOR LIFE

As an aid to integrating this program into your daily life, the acronym: **B.E. S.U.P.E.R. F.I.T.** is being used to describe this "10-Step Program".

The letters in each word remind you of the steps you will need to take each day to BE SUPER FIT and to THRIVE in a state of on-going wellbeing.

Each of these 10 steps works together in a holistic, synergistic way. They **ALL** help each other. If you leave any step out, you set up the potential for the "Weak Link" phenomena in which the whole program could be compromised.

What is the "Weak Link" phenomenon? Why is it important for you to include all 10 steps in your daily routine?

A chain is as strong as its weakest link. Take out one or two LETTERS in the phrase: BE SUPER FIT and you'll see what it means. **It takes all 10 steps to be SUPER FIT!**

B: BE IN COMMUNITY

We humans have been around for millions of years. Our success is unrivaled because we are the most social of all creatures. The motto of our human species: All for one, and one for all.

Our very power, as human beings, lies in community, cooperating, and sharing our knowledge. Just look at the Internet to see what this sharing looks like!

As the poet John Dunne once wrote, *"No man is an island unto himself."* Biochemically, it is known that when people get together, pain-killing endorphins are released and is the "feel good" neurotransmitter serotonin. That is, being with other people can boost our spirits and ***release a flood of feel-good painkillers***.

What are the life-affirming benefits of humanity, in community? They are many! When you join with others "in community" by attending social events, the theater, cultural events or participating in a group discussion, you diminish the health impacts of stress, anxiety, depression and loneliness.

Here's a story that will help you understand what I mean by life-affirming benefits. For example, serotonin is the major "feel good" chemical or neurotransmitter in your brain.

It is a medical fact that if someone gives a gift to someone else, the donor's serotonin level spikes. In addition, the recipient's serotonin level spikes. And, here's the part that directly benefits you...if someone is observing this action, say even from 100 feet away, his or her serotonin level will spike!

What does this say about the human COMMUNITY? That is literally biochemical proof of the commonality of mankind.

Could it be that what we have in common is our biochemical ability to automatically lift each other toward health and well-being when we share joy, happiness and good-will?

This is a BIG thought. Take a moment to let it sink in.

Is this why community is so important to us? The number one problem that sociologists and psychologists tell us that they are seeing, in every day modern day society, is lack of community.

This is the heart of it. Why is there an increase of stories related to stress, anxiety, depression and suicide reported in the daily news? Is there a common denominator? When asked: *professionals will tell us that 90% of the root cause of stress, anxiety, depression and suicide is due to the lack of community*. This erosion of community is happening around the world.

A final positive note, remember that music, laughter, and funny movies also provide connection to the greater human community. These too will lift your spirits.

E: EXERCISE AT AEROBIC LEVELS

In the 1960's, the world renown Dr. Kenneth Cooper was asked to train NASA astronauts for the world's first moon landing. They had to be in impeccable physical fitness for that 2-week sojourn. In his quest, Dr. Cooper asked the question: What really is fitness? In finding the answer, he made one of the greatest medical breakthroughs of the 20th century.

What was that breakthrough? That all exercise is not equal. One type of exercise needs oxygen, the other does not. So he coined two words to describe this: Aerobic [with oxygen] and Anaerobic [without oxygen] - such as lifting heavy weights.

Most of the medical benefits, Dr. Cooper showed, are from Aerobic exercise and most of these benefits relate to the **cardiovascular system**. This is good news because cardiovascular disease is the number one killer in the U.S.

So, if you want to do the minimal amount of aerobic exercise, <u>set aside 5-20 minutes every other day and you'll get most of the benefits</u>.

These <u>whole-body</u> health benefits include:

1. Strengthening the ventricles of the heart.
2. Lowering the bad LDL cholesterol.
3. Raising the good HDL cholesterol.
4. Preventing hardening of the arteries.
5. Boosting cell sensitivity to Insulin.

In addition, aerobic exercise has many mental benefits including the relief of stress, anxiety, and depression because it releases the "feel good" neurotransmitters: serotonin, dopamine, and endorphins.

EXPERIENCE A NATURAL HIGH

What this means for you is that by doing a minimum of 20 minutes of aerobic exercise each day, you can be put into the most POSITIVE state of mind. In addition, endorphins are the **PAIN-RELIEVING** neurotransmitters. Endorphins are the world's greatest natural painkillers.

Endorphins are **200 times** more powerful than morphine as a painkiller. Endorphin release occurs whenever you reach a **continuous level of aerobic exercise for a minimum of 20 minutes**.

And there is more to this story. You have Mother Nature's Whole Pharmacy inside your body. It's your own personal pharmacopoeia, free of charge. Without a prescription, you can evoke the entire pharmacy that Mother Nature gave you.

As a final point here, in addition to releasing serotonin and endorphins, aerobic exercise will also stimulate the production of the neurotransmitter dopamine in your brain.

Dopamine is the #1 neurotransmitter for motivation and GOAL SETTING. Whether at work, or on special projects, you want this neurotransmitter working on your behalf. **So to get motivated, get aerobic!**

WHAT *EXACTLY* IS AEROBIC EXERCISE?

This is what it is not. It is NOT weight lifting, golf, tennis, or even football. It is not a stop and start activity.

How do you reach aerobic levels each day? The key word here is CONTINOUS.

Aerobic exercise means the **continuous** use of oxygen for 20 minutes every day (or every other day, at a minimum). Aerobic exercise includes the following activities:

• fast walking

• running

• jogging

• bicycling

• swimming

The key idea here is to choose one activity and to do it non-stop for 20 minutes. My favorite is fast walking because I can do it anywhere.

AEROBIC WALKING IS KNOWN AS *"THE PERFECT EXERCISE"*.

How can you tell when you've reached aerobic levels through fast walking? The simple test is this: when you walk anywhere – even at a shopping mall – you will reach the point where you are barely able to talk to a friend while walking. That is, you will feel a bit breathless. You can still have a conversation, but it takes a bit of effort to talk.

S: STRETCH FLEXIBILITY AND CORE EXERCISES

To be SUPER FIT it's important to have a healthy mind, body and spirit. Body, mind and spirit are all connected. The fundamental axiom, body, mind and spirit is something that everyone involved in holistic medicine agrees upon.

Flexibility is especially important for **seniors** and people recovering from illness or injury. So any type of yoga, Pilates, core and flexibility exercise is important. You can do these exercises at home or at a gym. At home, you can use common household props as a stretching aid such as exercise balls and even simple rubber tubing.

If there is a chair, take a second to use it as an aid for stretching. If there is a wall, extend each arm up and stretch against the wall. In other words, you can use common ordinary everyday things like chairs and couches for stretching and flexibility.

When I take my dogs out for a daily walk, I even use the back bumper of the car — with the dogs patiently watching me — as a stretching prop while I do a few minutes of stretching before driving home.

All of these exercises automatically reduce STRESS in your body, while building your core strength. This is another simple way to boost your Immune System, on a daily basis, and acts as a personal health insurance policy to maintain or improve your good health.

The bottom line: when you use stretching exercises to gain flexibility and take stress away, you automatically help strengthen your body's IMMUNE SYSTEM. This helps you stay fit and healthy for life.

Is it possible to live a life where joy and joyfulness is within easy reach? **YES**, if you design your life to make it that way. Here's the goal: every single moment of life, on every single level, you want to keep stress to an absolute minimum. On the positive side, search out pleasurable activities such as massage, community events; aerobic; core and flexibility exercises; and, natural, unprocessed, nutrient-dense foods.

What these stress-free things have in common is that they help **turn off the mind**. They help shut down the stressful, negative thinking of the mind and they help shut down depression. In the process, you will find yourself so engaged in the activity that you have chosen, that it's almost impossible to conjure up a negative thought.

In addition, and again on the positive side, you will be releasing the powerhouse of **endorphins**, **serotonin** and **dopamine**. Working together, these three life-affirming neurotransmitters create a very powerful ally for your Immune System.

U: UNDERSTAND YOUR LIMITS. SAY "NO" TO DISTRACTIONS

Right now, what is most important to know is that the more a person is focused on a GOAL, the less they are going to be distracted by the demands of ordinary life.

For example, the following is a metaphor from sports, which you can apply to your own life.

The great sports medicine psychologist Dr. Jim Loehr began his career by studying two classes of athletes. The first were athletes of incredible talent and skill. The other, were athletes of lesser ability. He was perplexed by his observation that, in many cases, the athletes of **lesser** ability beat the athletes of **greater** ability and talent.

He asked why. The answer was found on the tennis court. In a typical match, the athletes of greater ability were easily distracted. The crowd, the noise, the discursive thoughts going through their minds, the negativity of self-criticism all swelled up like a volcano inside of them.

By contrast, the more mediocre athletes used the 20 seconds of downtime in between plays to create their own ritual. Some would never look at the crowd, or they would bounce the ball two or three times of twirl their tennis racket. They would stay in the zone of inward focus. The ritual each chose was to guarantee the locking in of a focused state, without negativity, without distractions, without discursive thoughts.

Then, upon serving the ball, their mind would be totally clear and focused and their natural talents would shine forth.

So how does this apply to you?

There will be many distractions in your life, just like those of the superstar athletes. So what is the antidote? Create your own life-affirming rituals for everyday living.

These might include **affirmations** during meals to affirm that the food will nourish your body and keep you in perfect health. They might be rituals to keep you focused whether at work, our in public, or at home. These rituals should always be framed in the affirmative.

ACTION: CREATE A LIST OF AFFIRMATIONS

Imagine waking every morning to a radio program or CD that begins with the sound of gentle surf at the ocean's edge. Then a clear, calm voice speaks to you. When you hear the voice, you begin to smile. Smiling changes your body chemistry and helps you absorb this message:

"Good morning and this is a good morning for you. This is the most important day in your life because it is now. Yesterday is then. Tomorrow is when. This day is now. You can use it and be it howsoever you desire. To do this, think of the most important act you can accomplish today. Think of it now. Now see yourself achieving that act or action, doing it easily and effortlessly, with positive results. Feel yourself doing it now."

Now say this to your mind:*

This day, I am stronger.

This day, I have greater physical and mental energy.

This day, I remain calm and relaxed.

This day, I think more clearly.

This day, I understand more of what I perceive.

This day, I have only constructive emotions.

This day, I feel great.

This day, I live in service and to help others.

This day, I assume authority and accept responsibility for myself.

This day, I perform my intended purpose.

This day, I am more than my physical body.

This day, I remember better who I am.

These affirmations are from the Monroe Institute CD, Morning Exercise. Htt;//www.monroeinstitute.org.

P: PACE YOURSELF, ESTABLISH RHYTHMS AND PATTERNS

Life is not linear. Life is day and night, work and rest, play and recovery. These rhythms of life are built into our very DNA, including 10,000 functions in our bodies.

These rhythms, or waves, are called **Circadian Rhythms**. Energy is expended. Energy is recovered. The heart beats, then rests.

In terms of "whole body" fitness, we should **make waves** every day. Our daily activities should include multiple waves of physical action and recovery. This is the lifestyle of the SUPER FIT.

Most people, in life, either in work or at play, expend too much energy for **long** periods of time, or too little. In the language of sports medicine, this is called either "over training" or "under training."

For the **TYPE A** workaholic personality, the term would be "over training." That is, they are constantly pushing themselves to do more, think harder, or work longer hours. This is **linear** activity. It is not actively creating **waves**. At the end of a long day, they might take time out for a workout, or perhaps once or twice a year, they might take time off for a vacation.

At the opposite extreme is the couch potato. The lifestyle of this person, perhaps basking in retirement, would be called "under training." It is also **linear**. This person is also not makes **waves** of action and recovery throughout the day. In both cases, the key word to apply here would be BALANCE.

For every energy expenditure, there should be an **equal and proportional** recovery time. The "**Golden Rule**" of sports is this: <u>**over training is worse than undertraining**</u>.

Here's a good example of BALANCE. Let's say you exercise at aerobic levels for 30 minutes every day. You would then need a *minimum* of 30 minutes of recovery time. The recovery time might include: light stretching, yoga, massage, or other low-impact exercise. Even "doing nothing", such as sitting on a chair, could be used for recovery.

At the other extreme is the "weekend warrior" who works hard all week long, and then does **too much** exercise on the weekend. This would be called "**over training**" and is also **linear**.

It is **linear** because they fail to make **waves** throughout each day. In Nature, this wave action throughout the day is called *Sinusoidal Oscillation*.

In addition, the "**weekend warrior**" who runs a long race, such as a marathon, and then does not allocate enough time after the race for recovery, can create health risks such as evoking the body's cortisone stress response (which targets the Immune System), inflammation, and the production of too many free radicals.

Here again, recovery exercises such as light stretching, yoga, and massage would be beneficial.

Overall, the **major** measurement of fitness is not <u>how much</u> you can do, but <u>how quickly</u> you recover.

E: VITAMIN E AND OTHER SUPPLEMENTS

There are known foods and supplements that have a whole-body benefit. Some of them are quite common.

1. **Vitamin C with bioflavonoids**. Vitamin C is known as ascorbic acid. Vitamin C always needs its helpers, which are called co-factors. And these co-factors are the bioflavonoids. For example, in the white of an orange, right under the skin, there are over 200 bioflavonoids. In addition, the most prevalent protein of the body is called COLLAGEN and only Vitamin C can make collagen. You need collagen!

   Collagen forms the tight matrix of the body. It's the "white stuff" that makes up your body, not your muscles. And this tight matrix of collagen is one of the body's **major** defenses against the spreading of cancer, called metastasis.

   If you like, you can buy Vitamin C (500 mg) *with* bioflavonoids, and then buy, in bulk, a powdered Vitamin C to boost your intake to 1.5 – 2.5 grams a day.

2. **Zinc** Is needed for maximum skin protection against infection, and for wound healing. It also erases stretch marks due to childbirth, or rapid weight loss.

3. **Vitamin E plus selenium.** Most topsoil is deficient in selenium. It is known to work synergistically, that is, beneficially, with Vitamin E. It helps Vitamin E reach it's maximum benefit for the body.

Vitamin E is the number one antioxidant for fat soluble substances such as oils and it works to **prevent** their oxidation in the body. Vitamin E also has many protective effects on the cardiovascular system. Whenever you buy Vitamin E, make sure it includes selenium.

4. **Nutritional Yeast.** The old yeast of the past was called Brewer's Yeast. When it is "tweaked" for human benefit, it is called Nutritional Yeast. Nutritional Yeast is the latest, beneficial generation of Brewer's Yeast. Nutritional Yeast is **50 % complete protein**. If you are a vegetarian or vegan, you can get a high-quality protein by taking Nutritional Yeast. *It also has all of the B-vitamins including the most expensive one B-12, in high, almost* **MEGA** *doses.* In addition, it has 17 different minerals, including hard-to=get minerals like selenium, chromium, and zinc.

5. **B-12 Sublingual.** A special note for SENIORS only. The anemia of children is IRON deficiency. The anemia of seniors is B-12 deficiency, also known as pernicious (meaning deadly) anemia.

The root cause of this in **seniors** is the attenuation of a protein carrier in the stomach as *we age*. That means you could be taking plenty of B-12, but if you, in your senior years, don't have that "shuttle bus" protein to get it into your blood, it won't be absorbed.

To get B-12 into their blood quickly, **seniors should take it in pill form under the tongue**. When you put the B-12 sublingual tablet under your tongue, it will be *immediately* absorbed into your blood, totally bypassing your digestive system.

6. **Lecithin.** Lecithin is a wonderful supplement to take to power the thinking part of your brain. It is the raw material for the famous neurotransmitter called **ACH** (acetylcholine). Any person who "thinks" for a living needs HIGH levels of ACH.

ACH is very low in patients with Alzheimer's, Parkinson's and other problems of the brain which are called dementias.

SUPPLEMENTS WHICH RELIEVE STRESS:

The following are all non-prescription. You can use one or all, at the same time. They are foods [amino acids], vitamins, minerals, or herbs. Protein is made up of 20 amino acids. Two of these are included here.

1. **Calcium.** The #1 mineral for relaxation of the body and muscles is calcium. Without sufficient calcium, the muscles cannot relax. This is also true for stomach cramps. Calcium will also help relax stomach muscles.

2. **GABA.** An *amino acid* which helps relax the brain.

3. **Tryptophan** (or 5 HTP). An *amino acid* which triggers the "feel good" chemical, serotonin.)

4. **Melatonin.** The sleep hormone that is used for both stress relief and a good night's sleep. (A warm bath also stimulates melatonin production.)

5. **Alpha Lipoic Acid.** Helps reduce free radicals in the body.

6. **Magnesium.** A mineral and is in a class of its own. It is called "nature's Tranquilizer." In addition to relaxation, it has over 300 different functions that benefit the body.

7. **DHEA.** The antidote for the "grumpy old man" syndrome. It also has anti-aging benefits.

8. **Valerian.** A natural herb that has been in use for hundreds of years to aid sleep.

R: RELAXATION, BIOFEEDBACK, AND MEDITATION

HOW **BIOFEEDBACK TECHNOLOGY** AIDS RELAXATION:

Biofeedback technology is perfect for use as an aid to intense visual imaging and goal setting. The basic concept is that Mother Nature gave us many feedback systems in the body. For example, you're hungry or thirsty, so you'll eat or drink. Once that thirst or hunger is satisfied, that mechanism will shut-off.

Biofeedback technology such as that used by training centers such as the Monroe Institute, or devices offered by companies such as TheWildDivine or ChooseMuse offer a way to accurately track our progress in reducing stress. It boosts our confidence level every step of the way. It is a technology that people love.

Why? The key benefit of biofeedback technology is this: *whenever we relax or meditate, the machine will give us feedback to tell us if we are doing the right thing.* This constant feedback assures us that we are gaining the benefits we seek through relaxation.

There are three major types of biofeedback.

1. The first type of biofeedback machine is one that is attached to the scalp with a headband, called Electroencephalograph (**EEG**) and will monitor your brainwaves. As you relax, your brainwaves slow down.

2. The second type of biofeedback is the Electrocardiogram (**EKG**). You are rewarded when you slow down your heart.

3. The third type of biofeedback is called EMG. EMG refers to the muscles. This biofeedback technology is attached to your muscles. The machine will give you a feedback response when you slow down your brainwaves, your heart rate, or when

you relax your muscles. The machine will give you feedback either as a sound or a light to let you know that your body is relaxing. The more you relax and slow down your brainwaves to the alpha state, slow down your heartbeat or relax your muscles, you get a little "visual cookie," a little sound bite, or other sensory feedback as a reward.

Another way biofeedback works is through **Operant Conditioning.** It is a type of learning that impacts the body. Using biofeedback technology, you are creating a learning style of body conditioning that B.F. Skinner, the famous psychologist, perfected. In short, you are learning how to slow down the functioning of your brain, heart, breath and muscles.

All of us have voluntary, conscious control over 640 muscles on the outside of the body. But what we do not have conscious control over is the *Autonomic Nervous System*. In a general way, it is the *Autonomic Nervous System* that bears the "hurricane" brunt of stress. When stress hits the heart, your heartbeat increases. When stress hits your brain, your brainwaves rise into a high-stress, beta state. **Operant Conditioning** then, through biofeedback, is a type of learning that, when consistently repeated helps us teach our *Autonomic Nervous System* how to relax. In a relaxed **ALPHA** state, we can encode positive images to help us reach our goals.

While biofeedback technology is a relatively new technology, it is important because it teaches us how to control the body's automatic stress response.

For example, in a crowded room, shouting out the word FIRE, even if there is no fire, will raise everyone's blood pressure. Operant conditioning through biofeedback teaches us to remain calm and centered.

Can you substitute meditation techniques? Yes, but here is why you might want to start with biofeedback technology.

With meditation, one never has actual proof that they're doing it right. By contrast, **the biofeedback technology's reward system is immediate proof from your body that you are doing it right**. It is proof that you are actually learning stress relief techniques.

If you want a confirmation that you're getting it right - go with the machine. It will give you positive feedback when you're doing the right thing. *As a confidence building factor, you want absolute proof that you are on the right track!*

Here's another benefit. When you use **EEG** biofeedback for your brain and learn how to quickly get into the alpha state, then you can also use that **ALPHA** state for intense visualization.

NOTE: Visualization works **best** when your brain is in an **ALPHA** state. When the brain is open and receptive, a suggestion, either [verbal] LEFT brain or [visual] RIGHT brain, will sink in the most successfully.

HOW MEDITATION WORKS....

Meditation is basically biofeedback without the machine. When used for goal setting, it does not give you clear confirmation that you achieved into an **ALPHA** state. If you want to make faster progress, start with confirmation of the **ALPHA** state through biofeedback. Then, if you like, make a transition to meditation techniques.

Another way to block negative thinking and get into a meditative state is through repetitive motion or sound.

Repetition of any thought, sound, or motion will bring you into an alpha or trance state over time. Examples might include a mantra repeated over and over. Or the repetition of a motion such as jogging or swimming. The very boredom of the repeated mantra, of the beat of your feet on the ground, or the swimming stroke, will drive you into an alpha state. In that state, you lose track of time.

When you lose track of time, you're in the **ALPHA** state. You don't notice the stress or pain of long-distance exercises - such as a marathon or long-distance swimming.

If you don't have access to a biofeedback machine, take a long walk and pay attention to your feet, because the repetitive sound of your feet on the ground – shhhh, shhh, shhh – will drive your mind into an **ALPHA** state.

NOTE: Meditation itself is stress release, as I mentioned, but don't stop there. Use that **ALPHA** state for conscious visualizations and suggestions about feeling **great**, being in **perfect** health, being SUPER-FIT, because that's when positive suggestions will sink-in. As mentioned before, you can use either verbal or visual suggestions or affirmations. However, it has been proven repeatedly that the intense **EIDETIC** method of visualization works the BEST.

HOW WE ACQUIRE NEW HABITS....

One form of learning is called **Imitation**. You mimic the actions of others. A child learns how to mimic the actions of their parents. An athlete watches the actions of Olympic level performers and tries to imitate the actions they see.

A second form of learning is **Classical Conditioning** discovered by Pavlov. I go into the kitchen - My dog associates that movement with food and begins to salivate.

The third form is **Operant Conditioning**. A child is good, and they get a reward. They get a reward for doing the right thing. A dog follows a command and they get a reward.

In each case the behavior is shaped by constantly rewarding the good behavior. In general, **Operant Conditioning**, using biofeedback technology shapes "inside" behavior; those things that happen "automatically" inside of your body.

To reduce stress, the key learning method is **Operant Conditioning**. _It should be directed inward, toward the visceral organs, and the Autonomic Nervous System_. Why? Stress happens really fast. Before you know it, it impacts the visceral organs and the autonomic nervous system inside the body. However, with practice, you can control this yourself.

F: FOODS THAT KEEP YOUR BODY SUPER FIT

Let's begin with digestive basics.

After any illness that requires antibiotics or surgery, it is mandatory that you follow an eating and lifestyle plan such as **23Ingredients**, and/or take one capsule of _Probiotic Acidophilus_ daily for two weeks to re-establish the friendly bacteria in your Gastrointestinal Tract [**GI**]. For example, Nature's Bounty Probiotic Acidophilus does not have to be refrigerated, and costs around $7 for 100 capsules. There are more expensive brands, however, this works just fine. After two weeks, you can return to one capsule a week, for life, which is sufficient.

And there's more news. At age 60, on average, 60% of your digestive juices are gone. At age 50, approximately 50% are gone. Whatever your age, it's important to pay close attention to what you eat and in what order. At each meal, you should start first with protein. In addition, at mealtimes you need to avoid diluting the digestive juices in your stomach with water, coffee, tea, soup, wine or beer. Furthermore, avoid upsetting the **Osmotic Balance** with too much sugar, salt, or unripe fruit because it may bring on a sudden, unwelcome bout of diarrhea.

As a rule of thumb, all liquids should be enjoyed up to 30 minutes before a meal, or at least 30 minutes after. If necessary, you can take digestive aids such as:

1. Hydrochloric acid (HCL) to digest protein in your stomach.
2. Ox bile to digest fats and oils in your liver.
3. Pancreatic enzymes to help digest carbohydrates.

You can buy these separately, or combined as one digestive pill. **These are all non-prescription.**

For those on the SUPER-FIT program, the **23Ingredient eating and lifestyle meal** supports your mind, body and spirit because it is:

1. Anti-inflammatory
2. Antioxidant
3. Avoids highly refined carbohydrates

This **eating and lifestyle** meal is the opposite of a highly refined carbohydrate diet, which is inflammatory. The NEW diet uses good fats as its fuel. It greatly lowers your carbohydrate intake, while at the same time, giving you a tremendous variety and choice of foods that you can eat.

For example, for protein, you can eat any type of beef, chicken, fish, milk or eggs. You can also enjoy any type of nuts. For carbohydrates, choose any type of vegetable or fruit that you like, and **use good fats** like butter, olive oil, avocado oil, coconut oil, coconut butter, high fat sour cream, high fat yogurt, high fat cheeses, nuts, and nut butters.

If possible, your diet should also include two known and powerful antioxidant spices such as turmeric (found in curry) and ginger.

What is absent from this diet are large amounts of highly refined carbohydrates such as overcooked pasta, breads, cakes, cookies, donuts, or pies.

NOTE: Please avoid stay away from carbonated sodas. Why? Because almost all sodas have high amounts of fructose corn syrup. The problem is that the body is not able, metabolically speaking, to handle high fructose corn syrup. Food or beverages with high fructose corn syrup will create additional health problems for cancer and heart patients alike.

The **eating and lifestyle meal** described in this book is particularly strong in focusing on anti-inflammatory grain-free foods, and also beneficial foods that are known as antioxidants - scavengers of free-radicals.

What are "free-radicals"? Free radicals are molecules in your body that cause extensive damage to all cells of the body. For athletes, "free-radicals" also come additionally, from intense exercise such as training for and running a marathon.

Antioxidants that work well to mop up the free-radicals of athletes also go to work inside cancer patient to mop up the free radicals created by radiation and chemotherapy.

The damage caused by free radicals in your body is indiscriminate. Think of each free radical molecule like a "bull in a china shop." Every cell in your body is at risk of damage.

Your job is to mop up the free-radicals each day by using **antioxidants found in fruits and vegetables, and** red wine, spices such as turmeric, ginger, and cinnamon, and super vitamins such as alpha lipoic acid, and Vitamin C with bioflavonoids.

Why do you need to mop them up? Free-radicals cause damage to your DNA which may mutate into a cancer. Free-radicals also attack your body's "energy factory" - the Mitochondria. Ironically, while processing glucose [from carbohydrates] the Mitochondria produce both energy and "smoke". The "smoke" is the free radicals that, in turn, will attack the Mitochondria in your cells.

Again, like a "bull in a china shop", free-radical molecules will bump into, and damage everything they come into contact with.

As a final note, consider adding these health and longevity boosters to your daily meals.

2 TBSP Oat Bran (for stool formation)

½ TBSP Wheat Bran (for internal cleansing)

1 TBSP Lecithin (supports the brain and heart)

1 TBSP Nutritional Yeast (rich with full-spectrum B vitamins including B-12. Note to seniors: please take B-12 sublingual, under the tongue.)

NOTE: A cow has four stomachs and up to 200 pounds of bacteria for digestion. A mountain gorilla consumes green vegetation all day long. By contrast, t*he human digestive system can only extract a small amount of nutrients, 5% to 15%, from a raw vegetable salad.* **So follow the 23INGREDIENTS eating and lifestyle meal - designed for humans!**

THE POWER OF PROTEIN

Most important, to be SUPER FIT is to build up and strengthen your body as fast as possible. The term used here is **Anabolic**, meaning, to build up the body. *And what builds up the body the fastest is protein.*

The word protein means "of first importance", because protein makes up your muscles, your bones (95% of your bones are made up of protein; 5% calcium), your enzymes, your antibodies, your cartilage, tendons and ligaments. Your whole body and your whole body chemistry are dependent upon protein.

One protein that satisfies these criteria perfectly is the common cage-free EGG. The egg holds the **"gold"** standard for protein.

Eggs are usually sold for about $3.50 a dozen. <u>The egg white, called albumin, has a protein rating of 100%</u>. All other proteins like beef (about 82%), like chicken and fish (about 75%) are relative to eggs.

NOTE: By having the very best protein: albumin, which has the best spectrum of body-building anabolic amino acids, you can build up a SUPER FIT body as fast as possible. In addition, please remember that the antibodies of your own immune system are 100% protein.

In addition, the yolk of the egg is the only major food source for the essential Vitamin D-3. Vitamin D-3 is known as the "Sunshine Vitamin." It has over 20 functions including preventing cancer, especially cancer of the prostate gland. Use a supplement to make sure you daily dose of Vitamin D-3 equals 2,000 I.U. a day.

Because you want to keep your Immune System strong, your body needs high quality protein to stay strong. Eggs are the Gold Standard for protein, with a rating of 100%.

The best way to prepare eggs in order to avoid chemical denaturation, is to cook them **as minimally** as possible.

For example: I cook my 2 soft-boiled eggs for three minutes, cool them down and then crack each one open and scoop out the contents into a bowl with a spoon and stir. I season this "egg drop" soup with salt, pepper and a splash of soy sauce, and enjoy it, daily.

NOTE: Please do not hard boil eggs for 8-12 minutes, or overcook them if turning into scrambled eggs or an omelet, because this renders the egg white [albumin] as an inferior protein. The chemical process that destroys the hard-boiled egg's protein by heat is called denaturation.

NOTE: Some of the best fish in the world that contain essential fatty acid **Omega-3** are sardines [complete with skin and bones] from cold water sources. The Omega-3 is in the fish skin. One that comes to mind is *King Oscar* sardines from Norway.

Any fish or fish oil with a Nordic or Icelandic, name in the label is a good choice because these northern waters are some of the cleanest on earth.

Omega-3 is also referred to as "Vitamin F". Interestingly, Vitamin F is actually composed of both Omega-6 and Omega-3. Most oils from plant sources are loaded with Omega 6. When asked, I recommend a minimum of 2 grams a day of Omega-3 fish oil.

When something is designated as a vitamin, it means it is an essential nutrient for the body; lack of which — by definition — causes a major disease. So please make a special note to include a daily dose of Vitamin F. Omega-3 has two sub-fractions: DHA and EPA. DHA feeds your brain while EPA nourishes your body.

Omega-3 [2 grams daily] is a daily insurance policy and provides protection against age-related diseases such as Alzheimer's and Parkinson's Disease. It reduces inflammation in the body; feeds the brain; and boosts your "feel good" serotonin levels.

NOTE: Many nights, I enjoy (or share) a tin of *King Oscar* sardines from Norway which have 2.5 grams of Omega-3. When I'm not eating sardines, or to make sure I have a daily dose of 2 grams or more, I use one tablespoon of Carslon Fish Oil, or Barlean's Purifed Omega Swirl, which tastes lemon meringue pie. Delicious!

Finally, there is less worry about mercury contamination in **cold-water** sardines, because the waters of the far north are some of the cleanest waters in the world. As well, sardines are near the bottom of the food chain, so few toxins concentrate in these fish.

So, use these BE SUPER FIT guidelines for food to boost your mood, your energy, and most important, your health.

I: IMAGINING YOURSELF AS SUPER FIT

Around 1948, at MIT, Dr. Norbert Weiner, one of the founding fathers of computers, coined the term **Cybernetics**, which comes from the Greek language and means "goal setting". His major insight was the capacity of the human mind to focus on a target or a goal. It's obvious, if we just look around at the whole human story, there are incredible achievements as a result of incredible goals in all fields of human endeavor and consciousness.

However, if that mechanism is blocked in any way, it may cause personal frustration - call it stress.

On a practical level, the way **Cybernetics** works is this...

We can act actually program our mind for the goals that we want to achieve. The new information in neurology is that we can program both the LEFT brain (verbal) and the RIGHT brain (visual). People who are more left brain, of course, will favor verbal programming. People who are more visual, will favor visual programming. The ideal, of course, would be to be able to do both because the left and right hemispheres are connected by a bridge of consciousness called the Corpus Callosum.

When programming your mind with a new goal, **the secret is to always see the END result first, as already done, a fait accompli, finished! That is, see yourself as SUPER FIT**.

The reason for this is because there is a phenomenon of very intense visualization, called Eidetic vision. Using Eidetic imagery, your nervous system will automatically incorporate this vision into every cell of your body.

What does this mean for you?

The basic technique for visualization and goal setting is to do it in a relaxed ALPHA state which, incidentally, also decreases your stress-related cortisone levels, while strengthening your Immune System.

Visualization works! For example, in the word of sports, it is known that if you have two groups of athletes, whatever the sport, and one group practices for one hour, and the other group practices for a half-hour but visualizes for the other half, the group that visualizes actually does better than the group that doesn't.

On a practical level, it's important to remember that your Eidetic vision sinks in best when your mind is in a relaxed **ALPHA** state. If you try to program yourself and do visualization during the normal conscious **BETA** state, your conscious mind just keeps challenging it. The mind is too critical, too analytical. The conscious mind will constantly say "No, you can't do this!" It will constantly challenge you.

Let's say you are in a BETA state and tell yourself: "I'm going to be the best player!" Your mind will constantly, logically challenge it. Your conscious mind will remind you that you might make a mistake, or that there are other good players, and so forth.

So, you need to drop into an ALPHA state to transcend your conscious, critical mind; that's the way Mother Nature works. That's why so many people are trapped. They just keep using LEFT brain logic. Logically, they are correct, so they don't take chances. Mother Nature says you've go to jump the gun and go to the end result, and then emblazon that image in your mind while in a relaxed ALPHA state.

The goal sinks in during the ALHA state. The key is to do that visualization as often as possible. Then engage as many senses (touch, sight, sound) as possible to support this visualization. Create a ritual around this goal, practicing multiple times a day.

Remember: your frontal cortex (the conscious mind) will keep challenging it. So get into an ALPHA state, or go even deeper into THETA, go to a relaxed brain wave state that won't be challenged by your left brain's critical analysis or negativity.

Mother Nature isn't logical. Love isn't logical. She will support whatever you imagine....in a relaxed ALPHA state.

For example, imagine this: "Mother Nature loves me. Mother Nature supports me, every second. Mother Nature has made me perfect in every way."

We're talking on a spiritual, transcendental level here. On this level, the cybernetic mind, the goal-setting mind, kicks in. Suggestions, both verbal and visual, sink in.

The more intense the Eidetic Image, the more it will sink in. The more confidence you have in the process, the more it will sink in. The more senses you bring to the imaging, the more it will sink in.

Biochemically, what seems to happen is this: when you get down to the Alpha State, by definition you are OFF the Cortisone State. When you are in the Alpha State which is around 10 cycles per second, you're accessing the PARAsympathetic nervous system.

The Parasympathetic nervous system is the receptive YIN state, the state where the seeds will take to the Mother Earth. What you are planting are the positive images and suggestions. They will take hold, take root and grow.

If your body is in resistance, nothing will take. If you body opens up and relaxes and is receptive, the images will take hold and grow. In an ALPHA state, imagery is in the form of suggestion will take hold.

It's also well known that through this type of **self-hypnosis**, the image will go to every cell in the body.

Go with faith or confidence. Even if you don't believe it, do it anyway!

T: TOUCH, MASSAGE, AND SLEEP

The great writer and anthropologist Ashley Montague, wrote the first book ever on touch. The title: TOUCH. One of the most underestimated tools in the human therapeutic arsenal is **TOUCH** in all its forms and varieties. Oh, and incidentally, he also wrote a famous book called **The Natural Superiority of Women!**

At the University of Miami Medical School, for example, the Director of the Institute of Massage, Tiffany Fields, has been studying the therapeutic effect of massage on cancer patients. Her work shows that, in many cases, touch has hundreds of different benefits. Benefits include releasing endorphins and serotonin. In our society, however, still to this day, many people have a taboo against touching someone else. But touch is as basic as food and air to human beings.

On a practical level, you can eve do **SELF- MASSAGE**. And if you like, for less than $50, you could simply buy a massage machine. The kind I use is called HoMedics. The company has a whole line of very inexpensive massage machines. *When you get a massage from someone else, or you do self-massage, what happens is you reduce the cortisone levels.* Touch reduces the stress hormone levels, especially the hormone cortisone.

What is cortisone? Mother Nature gave us a present at birth. It's our incredible Immune Defense System. The key word is DEFENSE. So not only does our Immune System defend us against bacteria and viruses, it also defends the SUPER FIT body against cancer. **Even in medical textbooks, the name of this phenomenon is called the "Immune Surveillance Against Cancer."**

And the part of the Immune System that is important here are the T-cells, which originate in the Thymus. The Thymus is located just above your heart.

The T-cells that originate in the thymus are the body's police force. Their job is to keep cancer cells under control. The POLICE stations where T-cells hang out are the **lymph nodes**. T-cells are on constant police surveillance. They go around and around in the lymphatic vessels through the whole body, looking for cancer cells to control. Whenever there is a breakout of cancer cells, the nearest, local police station sends out the T-cell cops. It's that simple.

Your Immune System constantly checks for cancer regardless of how it is formed, whether it comes from chronic physical or emotional stress, constant fear or negative thinking, the sun's ultraviolet rays, or even environmental toxins such as pesticides. And what kills cancer cells? The T-cells that originate in your thymus. And the biggest KILLER of your T-cells is the stress hormone CORTISONE.

The stress hormone cortisone is released from the cortex, the outside of your adrenal glands. Your adrenal glands are your stress glands. And with long-term stress, massive amounts of cortisone are released from the cortex.

For those on the BE SUPER FIT program, the name of the game is to support your Immune System by not evoking the cortisone response.

To do this on a daily basis, here are three important steps to take:

1. Reduce your cortisone levels by reducing stress in all its forms and varieties, including negative thinking. Find and hold positive images in your mind.

2. Take Vitamin C with bioflavonoids to strengthen your Immune System.

3. Take the mineral, Zinc. Zinc is basic for the health of the skin, which is the body's first line of defense. A good skin without any breaks or lesions is important to prevent germs from getting into the body. Zinc also facilitates wound healing and prevents stretch marks.

SELF-MASSAGE

One big way to reduce stress is with daily massage. Massage is a "sleeper," in the sense that it is one of those things that is basically free. You can do self-massage 10 times-a-day, if you like, using any kind of oil. You don't need expensive oils. Any oil will do.

What kind of oils? These might include inexpensive vegetable oils that stay liquid at room temperature. Remember, you are not using this oil for consumption. It is for external use only. You can then wipe it off with a towel or take a shower. At some stores, specialty massage oil might be as high as $10 for one to two ounces. The choice is up to you.

Why should you use oil, as opposed to an oil free massage? Oil helps reduce friction, and thus enable a deeper level of massage.

SLEEP WHAT YOU NEED TO KNOW ABOUT SLEEP.

According to Dr Maas, of Cornell Medical School, the average American sleeps about 60% less than compared to 100 years ago. Today, everything is 24/7 and the lights of big cities never go out, and the noise never stops, causing a tremendous sleep deprivation problem.

Getting a good night's sleep is especially important because of the secretion during sleep of the master hormone called **HGH** (Human Growth Hormone). For those on the BE SUPER FIT program, **HGH rebuilds all of the protein structures of the body**, not only your muscles and bones, but also the antibodies of your Immune System.

As you might have noticed, one of the great mega themes of this book has been keeping the Immune System as close to 100% strong as possible. And the building blocks of the Immune System are protein, which is laid down under the influence of **HGH**.

Mother Natures produces **HGH** mainly during sleep, in just the amounts you need. The greatest pulse of HGH occurs just before you reach seven hours and fifteen minutes of **sleep**.

SUPPLEMENTS WHICH CAN BE USED AS SLEEP AIDS:

The following sleep aids are non-prescription. You can use one or all at the same time because they are foods: amino acids, vitamins, minerals or herbs.

1. **Calcium**. The #1 mineral for relaxation of the body and muscles is **Calcium**. Without sufficient calcium, the muscles cannot relax.

2. **GABA.** An amino acid which helps relax the brain.

3. **Tryptophan.** 5 HTP is an amino acid which triggers the "feel good" chemical, serotonin.

4. **Melatonin.** The "sleep" hormone that is used for both stress relief and a good night's sleep.

5. **Magnesium.** This mineral is in a class of its own. It is called "Nature's Tranquilizer." It has over 300 different functions in the body. For the cancer survivor, it is used for relaxation.

6. **Valerian.** A natural herb that has been in use for hundreds of years for sleep.

FAQ FREQUENTLY ASKED QUESTIONS

FAST FACTS ABOUT **23INGREDIENTS** AND YOU:

1. The 23Ingredients Meal is 70% fiber, 15% fat & 15% protein.

2. Choose high-fiber [soft and hard] vegetables and fruits.

3. Eat <u>two meals a day</u> within an 8-hour period [12-noon - 7pm]

4. Sleep 8 hours/day; add 3-4 hours "buffer" before and after sleep to let your body complete its daily "home repair".

5. Stay hydrated with water or tea in between meals.

6. Snack #1: Enjoy 1 tbsp coconut oil. [Zero insulin response].

7. Snack #2: Add 1 tbsp each oat & wheat bran to water, hot tea or coffee and eat with a spoon. [Zero insulin response].

THE BASICS:

There are three food groups: protein, carbohydrates and fat.

High quality protein is required by your bones, your 640 muscles, ligaments, tendons and all of your body chemistry. Did you know that your bones are 95% protein and 5% calcium.

Carbohydrates are converted into sugar [**glucose**] by your body. Did you know that your body can only store **700** calories of **glucose** in your liver, however **your brain only needs 120 calories** of **glucose** a day. This amount is the same as eating an average size apple and half a banana each day.

AVOID highly refined grains found in baked goods, packaged foods such as chips, rice cakes, or pasta, or used as a thickener in soups. Pulverized grains rapidly turn into sugar [**glucose**] which then spikes the Insulin. **Beer** is considered "liquid bread" because it rapidly converts to **glucose**.Your body turns excess glucose into fat and stores it in your hips, arms, breast and belly.

BAD Carbs: An overweight, obese or insulin resistant body can be a sign of a body fueled by highly refined carbohydrates. This may create a higher risk of high blood pressure, heart attack, stroke, obesity, insulin resistance and diabetes.

GOOD Fat. Make fat your fuel. When you eat good fats at each meal your body quickly shifts to a fat-burning machine. In addition, your brain and heart run 25% better when good fat, converted into ketone bodies, is the fuel.

FAQ FREQUENTLY ASKED QUESTIONS ANSWERED

Beans/Legumes. *What is the rational for not including beans in the 23Ingredients?* Legumes are also called beans. They have what is called **Phytic acid** which means anti-nutrient. Physic acid i**mpairs the absorption of iron, zinc and calcium and may promote mineral deficiencies.** They may knock out a lot of minerals and prevent their absorption by the body. Beans also have a **high Glycemic index**, meaning that it raises the blood sugar. The best strategy is to include more of your standard vegetables rather than legumes.

Wheat, Rice and Corn. *Is there a link between the future of grains and climate change?* - Eighty percent of food that is eaten around the world is based on three grains: wheat, rice, and corn. All three crops rely on predictable rain and temperatures. Rising temperatures, damaging floods and drought due to climate change all bring a higher risk of widespread failure to this global food crop. The future of food requires that we think differently about our food choices. The **23Ingredients** eating and lifestyle meal was designed with optimum health and the future of foods - perhaps grown in greenhouses - on a warmer planet, in mind.

Sour Cream and Yogurt. *What is the best work-around/replacement ingredient if I can't eat sour cream or yogurt?* <u>Sour cream or yogurt will give the meal a creamy, luxurious texture.</u> It makes eating that much more pleasurable. The simplistic alternative is just to increase the other good fats [lipids], salad dressing, for example.

Red Bell Pepper Seeds. *Are they safe to consume?* - Did you know that the study of Red Bell Pepper seeds is where **Vitamin C** was actually discovered.... from the seeds themselves! For a normal healthy digestive system there is no problem eating the seeds. However, if you like, just avoid the seeds, cut up the sweet red bell pepper into slices and eat them raw.

Cheese [High Fat]. Why were these four specific cheeses chosen for *23Ingredients*? - The **high fat** cheeses that we listed are personal preferences. The choices you make may be different due to your own taste and cheeses that are available to you. The goal is to **have as many of the good fats as possible.** By increasing the fat you have at mealtime, what you are actually doing is keeping the need for protein down to a minimum. We recommend an increase in the good fats, and a decrease the protein you chose - down to the **size of a deck of cards**, or about 3 oz of protein a day for each of the two meals.

Pickles and Fermented Foods. <u>Are pickles an option? What type? What quantity?</u> Pickles would be excellent. What you are doing is creating a double benefit for your Microbiome if you include raw sauerkraut, kimchi, pickles, or any live cultured fruits and vegetables in your meal. You're giving the Microbiome the best soluble fiber it needs to make many beneficial chemicals for your body. The bacteria in those foods are facto-bacteria so you are giving the good bacteria in the microbiome a "population pulse"... you are adding **trillions of good bacteria** in this way.

Ripe Fruit and Dry Fruit. *Why are orange [or bananas] and raisins paired?* It is subjective to your own tastes and availability. These were the choices I made. For example, all fruits have pectin. Pectin is a favorite food of your microbiome which quickly converts into a pro-biotic within 24-hours in your colon. If you like, you can substitute dates or figs instead of raisins.

Plant Oil vs Olive Oil. *What's better?* The bottom line is this: the two vitamins consisting of Omega 6 and Omega 3 should be about 4 to 1 or 1 to 1 ratio. They are both vitamins - vital to health. However the Omega 6 is inflammatory. Omega 3 is anti-inflammatory. We need both, however in the US, the typical American diet is inflammatory, with about a 100 to 1 ratio.

Lecithin. *Where does Lecithin fit in, or not? What type of lecithin? Soya?* Yes. Soy is a bumper crop in the U.S. and is widely available. Lethicin contains phosphatidylserine and phosphorylcholine fancy names for two chemicals that are really good for your brain. They keep your brain cells nice and flexible and pliable to enable nutrients to continue flowing into the cells. With aging, they become more rigid. Lecithin keeps them flexible.

Goat and Sheep Cheese. *Is goat or sheep cheese acceptable for those who are allergic to A1 protein (lactose intolerant)?* - **Yes**.

Animal Protein. *Why must 23INGREDIENTS protein be "animal" protein?* The general reasoning is this: Animal protein is a direct match with our human protein. For example, the animal protein in the recommended two soft boiled eggs is called albumin, the egg white. The albumin in the egg is also the most prevalent protein in your body. Albumin is used for osmotic balance in every cell in your body. The egg yolk is not protein, however, it offers your body about 30 other benefits. Note: Both eggs and sardines are rated 100% protein.

Animal Protein: Turkey *Does turkey have **Tryptophane?*** Yes. Tryptophan is one of the 20 amino acids that is found in all animal protein including turkey. Tryptophan is the amino acid which makes the "feel good/bliss chemical," brain neurotransmitter seratonin.

Food Combining. *Can I get complete protein through food combining?* Yes. You can get complete protein by combining grains and beans/legumes. However it is like a "Grade C" protein because it is not a direct match with your body. Those who practice food combining choose one from Group A [grains, for example] and one from Group B [beans/legumes] to create a meal that has all 20 amino acids found in complete protein.

You will get a complete protein, however it is like getting a grade of only 65 on an exam. That protein, even though it is complete and has all 20 amino acids, is totally different from the protein in your own body. With egg white [albumin] you are getting the exact spectrum that matches your own body.

NOTE: Food combining comes with certain risks. Whether the choice is to combine rice and beans in the West, or tabouli (tabbouleh) and hummus in the East, the glycemic load is too high. **It turns into sugar too fast in the body;** causes an **Insulin response** and, the corresponding **Metabolic Syndrome**.

The bottom line: beans [legumes] have anti-nutrients. However, around the world, for various reasons, people will use them for food combining because there are few or no animal products available where they live; or because of religious dietary restrictions. Hindus, for example, do not eat animal protein. People in some parts of the world may do "food combining" for economic reasons; they cannot afford animal protein.

Whatever the reason, those who food combine will sustain LIFE but it will also have three significant impacts:

1. It will increase the **Gylcymic** load and the **Insulin** response causing inflammation which correlates with the **Metabolic Syndrome**.

2. It will have anti-nutrients in the beans [legumes].

3. The protein that you get from food combining is a very inefficient way for children to grow strong bones - which are 95% protein, or for seniors to repair their own body after daily activity.

Metabolic Syndrome and Diabetes Syndrome. These are the issues that should concern seniors.

In 1980, at Stanford Medical School, Dr. Raven, Head of Endocrinology (the study of hormones) discovered a link, a constellation of traits: high blood pressure, obesity, cardio vascular disease, stroke, insulin resistance, and or full diabetes, and that they are all linked together.

At the time, Dr. Raven didn't know the cause. Two years later he worked out the cause: the hormone **Insulin**.

There is one, and only one food group, that really spikes the insulin - **highly refined carbohydrates**, especially cereal grains. Highly refined carbohydrates spike the insulin like crazy.

Your body can run on two kinds of fuel: **carbohydrates** or **good fats**. The carbohydrate-based-fuel is glucose (sugar) from a diet that includes products made from highly refined grains like wheat, rice and corn. It will keep you alive, but it is not the most efficient fuel. It provides quick energy, like burning wood, and is inflammatory.

When you use good fat, like avocados, olive oil and butter in the diet it serves as the primary fuel for the body. The good fat gives virtually zero insulin response.

When you choose **good fats** as your fuel at mealtime - the more you are choosing an anti-inflammation eating and lifestyle meal. **Fat is converted into ketone bodies.** Both your brain and your heart run 25% more efficiently on ketone bodies. In addition, when you choose good fats, what you are doing is undercutting the **Metabolic Syndrome**.

Nuts. *Which nuts are best?* Any kind of nut would be excellent. Avoid salted nuts. The best source of Omega 6 is nuts or nut butter. A small handful of nuts daily is part of 23INGREDIENTS.

Pumpkin? Sunflower? *Can I include these?* Yes.

Coconut Oil / Coconut Butter. *Is this a good fat?* Yes. Coconut oil is a good fat and dissolves in water without triggering your digestive juices. It has zero insulin response. This means that when you eat one tablespoon of **coconut oil**, it immediately dissolves in your body and becomes accessible as fuel. One tablespoon of coconut oil in between meals can also cut your cravings for snack foods. By contrast, **Coconut Butter** is the whole coconut with fiber. Use it like a gourmet treat. Scoop directly out of the jar and use as a high energy snack.

Mother Nature gave us three food groups. They are called the macro-nutrients. The three big ones are:

Protein. Protein means "of first importance" and includes the animal flesh, such as beef, chicken or fish, or any product from an animal such as eggs, milk, cheese or yogurt. The animal itself or the products. It has 20 different amino acids. Only protein can make your bones, muscles, ligaments and neurotransmitters. Protein supports bone growth in children. In seniors with active lifestyles, there will be wear and tear. The body cannot make new body tissue with fat or carbohydrates. <u>Protein is used for growth in children; in seniors, it is used for repair.</u>

What is the optimum amount? 3oz. of protein a day. Think of the size of a deck of cards, or a tin of sardines.

Good Fats. Fats are synonymous with lipids. Fats are the main components of tissues like brain, nerves and hormones. Fats come in two varieties: animal fat and plant fat. In a juicy steak or hamburger the juice is the fat. In plants, it's plant oils.

They come in three different varieties:

1. **Mono-unsaturated GOOD fats include olive oil, olives, avocado oil, avocados, and canola oil.**
2. **Saturated fats** can be filled with hydrogen. Avoid.
3. **Polyunsaturated fats** such as safflower, sunflower, sesame, and peanut oils are high in Omega 6.

Carbohydrates found in vegetables and fruit are called glucose. Glucose is a fuel for the body as is lactose from milk, and aslo fructose. Each of these: lactose, fructose, or glucose are all example of carbohydrates. Chose high-fiber fruits and vegetables. Avoid juicing. Avoid foods sweetened with fructose.

<u>Today, 80% of the world's calories now come from wheat, rice and corn.</u> **AVOID** highly refined grains that are turned into products such as chips, cookies, energy bars, cakes and pastries. Why? **They can spike your insulin** due to large amounts of **sugar (glucose) and very little or ZERO fiber.**

High fiber vegetables, like carrots, may taste sweet, however, functionally, **vegetables have a low glycemic rating** because they also have so much fiber. High fiber-rich foods slow down the process of absorption of sugar and avoids spiking the Insulin.

Fiber-Rich Fruits. *What are considered fiber-rich foods?* All fruits contain "fiber-rich" soluble and insoluble fiber. The biggest share of the soluble fiber would be in fruit. It's called "pectin". Pectin-rich fruits including apples, blueberries and strawberries are a favorite soluble fruit for the microbiome. Fiber-rich foods slow down the absorption of sugar by the body.

By contrast, fruits such as melons and watermelon - called "juicy or succulent fruits" - **have a tremendous amount of sugar and very little fiber.** So, use a very small amount. Juicy fruits are mainly sugar in liquid form. Plums, peaches, melons and oranges all have the fruit sugar called fructose. Many juicy fruits are bred by commercial interests to contain a high amount of sugar. A small slice is OK. **Remember to avoid drinking your fruit.**

Fructose. In the U.S. there is a bumper crop of corn. High fructose sugar is produced from corn. The result is that fructose undercuts the import of sugar from other sources because fructose - as a sweetener - is cheaper. <u>Because of its lower cost, fructose is put into many foods to boost their sugar content.</u> Too much fructose, absorbed too fast, as in juice drinks, <u>spikes the insulin</u>.

Lemon Juice. *Is there a limit to how much pure lemon juice one can use, throughout a day in hot water? Does it create or upset the PH ... acid v. alkaline balance?* There is no concern with too much acid because the body has a buffer mechanism in the blood to control the amount of acid delivered to it. The main issue related to using a lot of lemon juice (or apple cider vinegar), is that it may wear away the teeth enamel over time.

Turmeric. Is powdered turmeric, ginger, paprika, cayenne, onion, pepper, cinnamon, nutmeg, allspice acceptable if used sparingly e.g. 1/8 of a teaspoon? Certain spices and herbs like turmeric which has curcumin, is a very powerful anti-oxidant and anti-inflammatory.

What the **23INGREDIENTS** Meal Planner means for YOU is that you don't have to be Spartan.

If you like, enjoy a little red wine, a variety of spices, including turmeric, along with 70%+ dark chocolate, coffee and green tea each day.

Ready to start the 21-Day Challenge

START HERE:

23INGREDIENTS Menu Planner & 21-Day Workbook

Please send your comments and feedback to:
hello@10TRAITS.org

Made in the USA
Las Vegas, NV
01 November 2022

58575883R00042